ASTHMA-WHOLESOME EATS

Nourishing Recipes for Lasting Relief

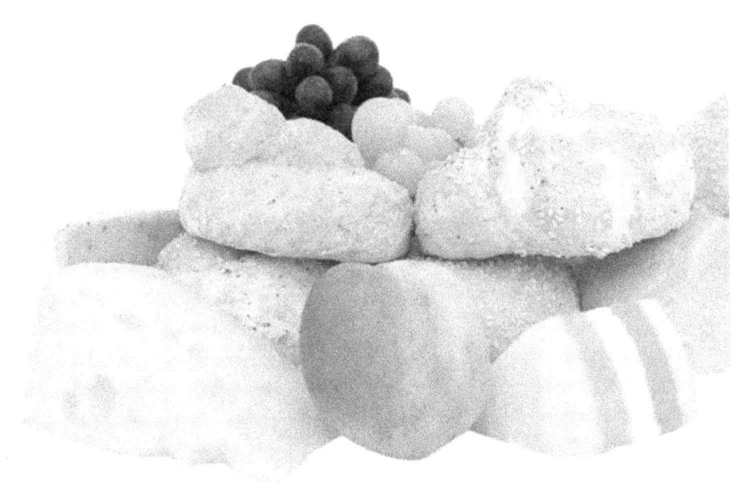

Susan Ribble

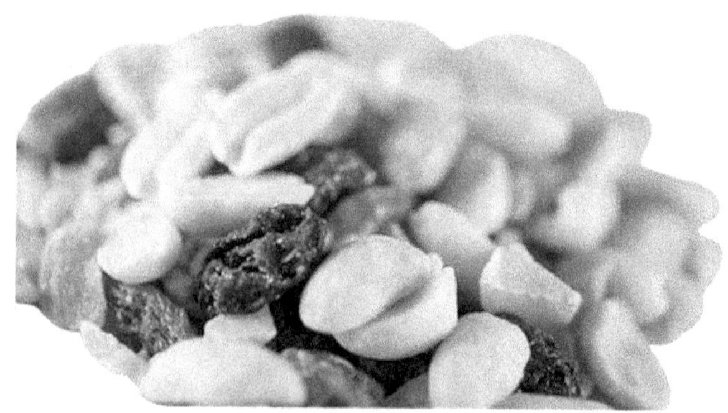

TABLE OF CONTENTS

INTRODUCTION

Welcome to "Asthma-Wholesome Eats: Nourishing Recipes for Lasting Relief," your essential guide to breathing easier through the power of nutritious food. If you or a loved one is among the millions of people affected by asthma, you know how this chronic condition can impact every aspect of life. But did you know that what you eat can play a crucial role in managing asthma symptoms and improving your overall well-being?

Asthma is a condition characterized by inflammation and narrowing of the airways, leading to breathing difficulties, wheezing, and coughing. Common triggers include allergens, pollution, respiratory infections, and even stress. While medication and lifestyle changes are vital for managing asthma, emerging research highlights the significant influence of diet on respiratory health.

The foods you choose can either exacerbate or alleviate asthma symptoms. Nutrient-rich foods can reduce inflammation, strengthen the immune system, and promote overall lung health. Conversely, processed foods, additives, and certain allergens can worsen asthma symptoms. By focusing on wholesome, nutritious ingredients, you can create meals that not only taste delicious but also support your respiratory health.

In this book, you will discover a treasure trove of asthma-friendly recipes designed to nourish your body and help you breathe easier. From antioxidant-rich fruits and vegetables to anti-inflammatory herbs and spices, each recipe is crafted with ingredients known for their beneficial effects on asthma.

Embark on this culinary journey with me, and learn how to transform your diet into a powerful tool for managing asthma.

CHAPTER ONE

Understanding Asthma

Asthma is a chronic respiratory condition characterized by inflammation and narrowing of the airways, which can lead to difficulty breathing, coughing, wheezing, and shortness of breath. Understanding the mechanisms, triggers, and management strategies for asthma is essential for effectively controlling the condition and improving quality of life.

What Happens in Asthma?

Asthma involves several key processes within the airways:

Inflammation: The lining of the airways becomes swollen and inflamed, which narrows the air passages and makes breathing difficult.

Broncho constriction: The muscles surrounding the airways tighten, further constricting the flow of air.

Mucus Production: Increased production of mucus can clog the airways, exacerbating breathing difficulties.

Common Symptoms

Asthma symptoms can vary in intensity and frequency, but common signs include:

- Shortness of breath
- Wheezing (a whistling sound when breathing)
- Chronic coughing, especially at night or early morning
- Chest tightness or pain

Triggers

Asthma can be triggered by various factors, which may differ from person to person. Common triggers include:

- Allergens: Pollen, dust mites, pet dander, mold, and certain foods can trigger allergic reactions and asthma symptoms.
- Irritants: Tobacco smoke, air pollution, strong odours, and chemical fumes.
- Respiratory Infections: Colds, flu, and other respiratory infections.
- Physical Activity: Exercise-induced asthma.

- Weather Conditions: Cold air, humidity, and sudden temperature changes.

- Emotional Stress: Strong emotions such as stress or excitement.

Types of Asthma

Asthma can be classified into different types based on the underlying cause and the nature of the symptoms:

- Allergic Asthma: Triggered by allergens such as pollen, dust mites, and pet dander.

- Non-Allergic Asthma: Triggered by irritants like smoke, pollution, or strong odours.

- Exercise-Induced Asthma: Triggered by physical activity.

- Occupational Asthma: Triggered by exposure to substances in the workplace.

- Childhood Asthma: Asthma that develops in children, often related to allergies.

Diagnosis and Management:

Medical Evaluation: Diagnosis of asthma typically involves a thorough medical history, physical examination, and lung function tests such as spirometer and peak flow measurements.

Treatment: Asthma management aims to control symptoms, prevent asthma attacks, and improve quality of life. This often involves a combination of medications, including long-term control medications (such as inhaled corticosteroids) and quick-relief medications (such as bronchodilators).

Lifestyle Modifications: Identifying and avoiding triggers, maintaining a healthy weight, quitting smoking, and staying physically active can help manage asthma symptoms and reduce the frequency of asthma attacks.

Asthma Action Plan: Individuals with asthma should work with their healthcare providers to develop a personalized asthma action plan. This plan outlines daily management strategies, steps to take during asthma attacks, and when to seek emergency medical care.

Importance of Monitoring:

Symptom Tracking: Regular monitoring of asthma symptoms, peak flow measurements, and medication use can help individuals and their healthcare providers assess asthma control and adjust treatment as needed.

Preventive Measures: By recognizing early warning signs of worsening asthma and taking preventive measures, individuals can reduce the risk of severe asthma attacks and hospitalizations.

Emergency Preparedness: Knowing when to seek emergency medical care is crucial for individuals with asthma. Severe asthma attacks require prompt treatment to prevent life-threatening complications.

Understanding asthma is essential for effective management and improved quality of life. By identifying triggers, following a personalized treatment plan, and staying vigilant about symptom monitoring, individuals with asthma can lead active, fulfilling lives while minimizing the impact of this chronic condition.

Collaboration with healthcare providers, adherence to treatment, and proactive self-management are key to successfully managing asthma and achieving long-term relief.

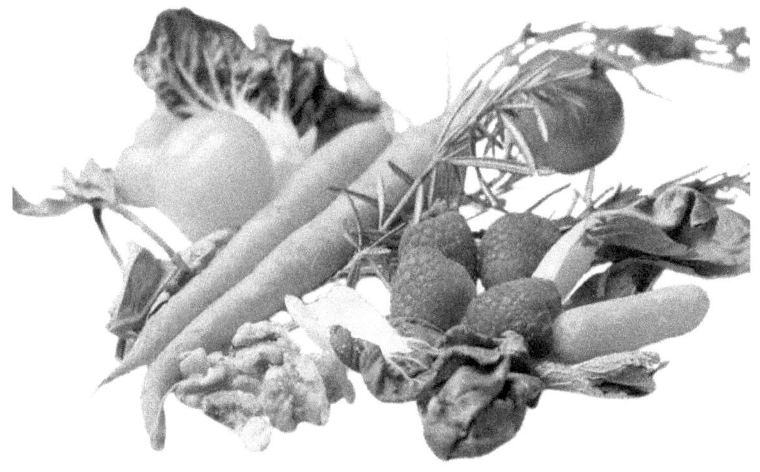

CHAPTER TWO

Essential Nutrients for Lung Health

The importance of respiratory health cannot be overstated. Our lungs are essential for the exchange of oxygen and carbon dioxide, crucial for sustaining life. Yet, factors such as pollution, smoking, and respiratory illnesses can compromise lung function. However, a well-balanced diet rich in essential nutrients can play a significant role in supporting lung health and function.

Vitamin C

One of the most well-known antioxidants, vitamin C, is vital for lung health. Its potent antioxidant properties help protect lung tissues from oxidative damage caused by pollutants and irritants. Vitamin C also plays a crucial role in the synthesis of collagen, a structural protein necessary for maintaining the integrity of lung tissue. Furthermore, vitamin C has been shown to reduce the severity and duration of respiratory infections by enhancing immune function. Citrus fruits, berries, kiwi, peppers, and broccoli are excellent sources of vitamin C.

Vitamin E

Another powerful antioxidant, vitamin E, is essential for protecting lung cells from damage caused by free radicals. By neutralizing these harmful molecules, vitamin E helps reduce inflammation in the lungs and promote respiratory health. Studies have shown that adequate intake of vitamin E is associated with a lower risk of developing chronic respiratory conditions such as asthma and chronic obstructive pulmonary disease (COPD). Nuts, seeds, vegetable oils, and leafy greens are rich sources of vitamin E.

Vitamin D

Often referred to as the "sunshine vitamin," vitamin D plays a crucial role in immune function and inflammation regulation, both of which are important for maintaining healthy lungs. Research suggests that vitamin D deficiency may be associated with an increased risk of respiratory infections and exacerbations of chronic respiratory conditions such as asthma and COPD.

Additionally, vitamin D has been shown to modulate lung function and reduce airway inflammation. Fatty fish, fortified dairy products, eggs, and sunlight exposure are primary sources of vitamin D.

Omega-3 Fatty Acids

Omega-3 fatty acids, found primarily in fatty fish like salmon, mackerel, and sardines, as well as in flaxseeds and walnuts, have potent anti-inflammatory properties that can benefit lung health. By reducing inflammation in the airways, omega-3 fatty acids may help alleviate symptoms of respiratory conditions such as asthma and COPD. Furthermore, omega-3 fatty acids have been shown to improve lung function and reduce the risk of respiratory infections.

Magnesium

Magnesium is a mineral that plays a crucial role in muscle function and relaxation, including the smooth muscles surrounding the airways. Adequate intake of magnesium is associated with improved lung function and reduced risk of asthma exacerbations.

Furthermore, magnesium deficiency has been linked to increased airway hyper reactivity and broncho-constriction. Nuts, seeds, whole grains, and leafy green vegetables are excellent sources of magnesium.

Selenium

Selenium is an essential trace mineral with antioxidant properties that help protect lung cells from oxidative damage. Studies have shown that selenium deficiency may be associated with an increased risk of asthma and other respiratory conditions.

Furthermore, selenium plays a crucial role in immune function, helping the body fight off respiratory infections. Seafood, Brazil nuts, poultry, and eggs are primary dietary sources of selenium.

Zinc

Zinc is a trace mineral that plays a crucial role in immune function and wound healing. Adequate intake of zinc is essential for maintaining optimal respiratory health, as zinc deficiency has been associated with an increased risk of respiratory infections and exacerbations of chronic respiratory conditions. Furthermore, zinc has been shown to have antiviral properties, helping to reduce the severity and duration of respiratory infections. Meat, shellfish, legumes, seeds, and nuts are excellent sources of zinc.

Quercetin

Quercetin is a flavonoid with potent antioxidant and anti-inflammatory properties that can benefit lung health. Studies have shown that quercetin supplementation may help reduce inflammation in the airways and improve lung function in individuals with respiratory conditions such as asthma and allergies. Quercetin is found naturally in foods such as onions, apples, berries, and green tea.

Essential nutrients play a crucial role in supporting lung health and function. Vitamins C, E, and D, omega-3 fatty acids, magnesium, selenium, zinc, and quercetin all contribute to maintaining optimal respiratory health by protecting lung cells from oxidative damage, reducing inflammation in the airways, and enhancing immune function.

By incorporating these key nutrients into a well-balanced diet, individuals can support their lung health and reduce the risk of respiratory issues. However, it is essential to consult with a healthcare professional before making any significant changes to dietary intake, especially for individuals with pre-existing medical conditions.

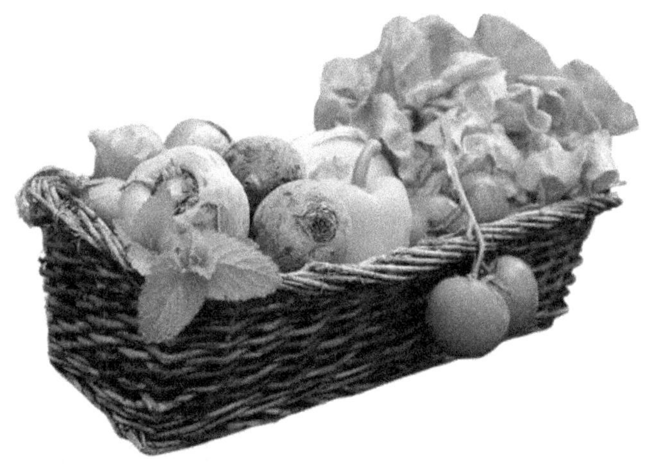

CHAPTER THREE

Super foods for Asthma Relief

Asthma, a chronic respiratory condition affecting millions worldwide, can significantly impact daily life. While medication is essential in managing symptoms, the role of diet in supporting respiratory health should not be underestimated. Super foods, nutrient-rich foods packed with vitamins, minerals, antioxidants, and anti-inflammatory compounds, offer promising benefits for individuals with asthma. In this chapter, we will explore the top 10 super foods for better breathing and creative ways to incorporate them into your diet for asthma relief

Top 10 Super foods for Better Breathing

Salmon: Rich in omega-3 fatty acids, salmon possesses potent anti-inflammatory properties that can help reduce airway inflammation and improve lung function in individuals with asthma. Regular consumption of fatty fish like salmon has been associated with a lower risk of asthma symptoms and exacerbations.

Berries: Blueberries, strawberries, raspberries, and blackberries are bursting with antioxidants, particularly flavonoids and vitamin C, which help combat oxidative stress and inflammation in the airways. These delicious fruits can help reduce the severity and frequency of asthma attacks.

Spinach: Leafy greens like spinach are rich in magnesium, a mineral known for its bronchodilator properties. Magnesium helps relax the smooth muscles of the airways, making it easier to breathe for asthma sufferers. Incorporating spinach into your diet can support respiratory health and reduce asthma symptoms.

Turmeric: This golden spice contains curcumin, a compound renowned for its anti-inflammatory and antioxidant properties. Curcumin has been shown to alleviate airway inflammation and improve lung function in individuals with asthma. Adding turmeric to your meals or consuming it as a supplement can provide relief from asthma symptoms.

Avocado: Avocados are packed with vitamin E, an antioxidant that helps protect lung cells from oxidative damage and inflammation. Vitamin E has been shown to reduce airway constriction and improve lung function in individuals with asthma. Including avocados in your diet can support respiratory health and reduce asthma symptoms.

Quinoa: A nutritional powerhouse, quinoa supplies ample magnesium and fibre, which collectively reduce inflammation and support gastrointestinal health, vital for asthma management.

Walnuts: Brimming with omega-3 fatty acids and vitamin E, walnuts curb airway inflammation and safeguard lung cells from oxidative stress, contributing to enhanced respiratory function.

Kale: Rich in vitamin C and antioxidants, kale aids in quelling airway inflammation, thereby facilitating smoother breathing and improved lung function in individuals with asthma.

Ginger: Gingerol, the bioactive compound in ginger, boasts potent anti-inflammatory and bronchodilator properties, offering significant relief from asthma symptoms and improving respiratory health.

Pumpkin Seeds: Packed with magnesium, zinc, and antioxidants, pumpkin seeds play a pivotal role in reducing airway inflammation and bolstering immune function, crucial for asthma management.

Creative Ways to Add Super foods to Your Diet

Are you ready to supercharge your meals and fuel your body with the goodness it craves? Say hello to the superheroes of nutrition – super foods! These powerhouse ingredients are bursting with vitamins, minerals, and antioxidants, offering a deliciously effective way to support your health goals, including managing asthma symptoms. But incorporating them into your diet doesn't have to be boring or complicated. Here are some creative and inspiring ways to add these nutritional superheroes to your meals:

Smoothie Bliss: Blend up a storm with a rainbow of fruits like berries, mango, and banana, then add a handful of nutrient-rich spinach or kale and a spoonful of chia seeds or hemp hearts for an unbeatable morning boost.

Salad Symphony: Transform your salads into vibrant works of art by tossing in a mix of super foods like avocado, pomegranate seeds, and toasted nuts or seeds. Drizzle with a homemade vinaigrette featuring super food ingredients like olive oil and apple cider vinegar for extra oomph.

Bowl Bonanza: Build your own Buddha bowl masterpiece with a base of quinoa or brown rice, then pile on the super foods – think roasted sweet potatoes, steamed broccoli, and creamy tahini dressing for a satisfying and nourishing meal.

Stir-Fry Sensation: Turn up the heat with a sizzling stir-fry loaded with colourful veggies, lean protein like tofu or chicken, and aromatic spices like ginger and garlic. Top with a sprinkle of sesame seeds or a drizzle of tamari sauce for an irresistible flavour explosion.

Snack Attack: Ditch the processed snacks and reach for wholesome super food options like air-popped popcorn sprinkled with nutritional yeast, crunchy kale chips, or energy balls made with dates, nuts, and cacao nibs for a sweet and satisfying pick-me-up.

Toast Toppers: Upgrade your morning toast routine by slathering on mashed avocado or almond butter, then layering on sliced strawberries, banana, and a sprinkle of cinnamon for a nutrient-packed start to the day.

Soup Spectacular: Warm up with a comforting bowl of soup brimming with super foods like lentils, kale, and turmeric. Get creative with your spices and seasonings to create a flavour-packed masterpiece that's as nourishing as it is delicious.

Oatmeal Oasis: Take your breakfast game to new heights with a bowl of creamy oatmeal topped with super food goodies like goji berries, toasted coconut flakes, and a dollop of creamy almond butter for a hearty and satisfying morning meal.

Dip Delight: Whip up a batch of homemade hummus or guacamole using super food ingredients like chickpeas or avocado, then pair with crunchy veggie sticks or whole-grain crackers for a nutritious and flavourful snack.

Super food Sweets: Indulge your sweet tooth with guilt-free treats like dark chocolate-covered almonds, homemade granola bars packed with nuts and seeds, or a decadent smoothie bowl topped with fresh fruit and shredded coconut for a delicious and nutritious dessert option.

With these creative and mouth-watering ideas, incorporating super foods into your diet has never been easier – or more delicious! So, why wait? Dive in and discover the endless possibilities of super food cuisine, and watch as your health and vitality soar to new heights.

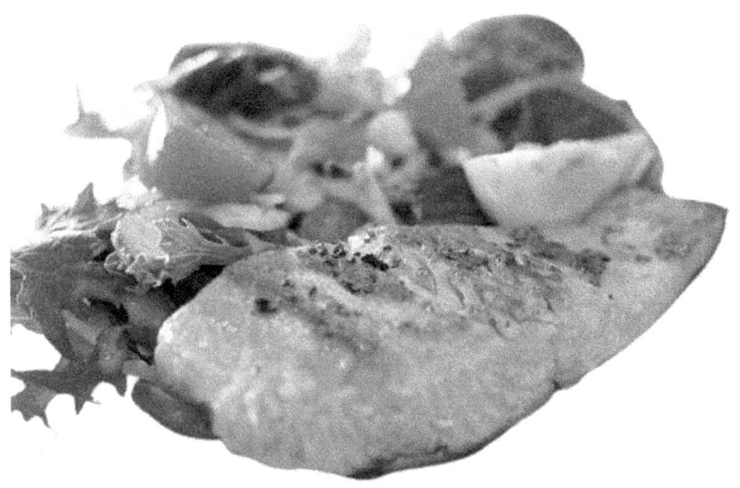

CHAPTER FOUR

Energizing Breakfasts

They say breakfast is the most important meal of the day, and for good reason. A nourishing morning meal not only provides the fuel your body needs to kick-start the day but also sets the tone for healthier eating habits throughout the day. From hearty oats to protein-packed smoothies, energizing breakfasts offer a delicious and nutritious way to power up your morning routine. In this essay, we'll explore a variety of morning meals guaranteed to energize your body and mind, setting you up for success from sunrise to sunset.

Hearty Oatmeal Creations

Oatmeal is a classic breakfast choice that's not only comforting but also incredibly versatile. Start your day right with a bowl of warm oatmeal topped with a variety of nutritious toppings:

Banana Nut Oatmeal: Top your oatmeal with sliced bananas, chopped nuts, and a drizzle of honey for a sweet and satisfying start to your day.

Berry Bliss Oatmeal: Mix fresh or frozen berries into your oatmeal, then sprinkle with chia seeds and a dollop of Greek yogurt for a burst of flavour and protein.

Pumpkin Spice Oatmeal: Stir canned pumpkin puree and a dash of pumpkin pie spice into your oatmeal, then top with toasted pecans and a sprinkle of cinnamon for a cozy autumn-inspired breakfast.

Protein-Packed Smoothie Bowls:

Smoothie bowls are not only delicious but also a convenient way to pack in nutrients and energize your morning routine. Blend up your favourite fruits and veggies, then top with crunchy granola, nuts, and seeds for added texture and flavour:

Tropical Paradise Bowl: Blend frozen mango, pineapple, and banana with coconut water, then top with sliced kiwi, shredded coconut, and a sprinkle of hemp seeds for a taste of the tropics.

Green Goddess Bowl: Blend spinach, kale, banana, and pineapple with almond milk, then top with sliced avocado, pumpkin seeds, and a drizzle of honey for a nutritious and refreshing breakfast.

Chocolate Peanut Butter Bowl: Blend frozen banana, cocoa powder, and peanut butter with almond milk, then top with sliced strawberries, crushed peanuts, and a drizzle of melted dark chocolate for a decadent and protein-rich breakfast treat.

Egg-cellent Breakfast Ideas:

Eggs are a versatile and nutrient-rich breakfast option that can be enjoyed in countless ways. Try these egg-cellent breakfast ideas to start your day off on the right foot:

Avocado Toast with Eggs: Top whole-grain toast with mashed avocado and a fried or poached egg, then sprinkle with red pepper flakes and a squeeze of lemon juice for a simple yet satisfying breakfast.

Vegetable Frittata: Whip up a vegetable-packed frittata using eggs, spinach, bell peppers, onions, and feta cheese, then slice into wedges and enjoy hot or cold for a nutritious and filling breakfast option.

Egg Muffins: Make a batch of egg muffins by whisking together eggs, chopped vegetables, and cheese, then pouring into muffin tins and baking until set. Enjoy them hot or cold for a protein-packed breakfast on the go.

Energizing breakfasts are the key to starting your day off on the right foot and fueling your body for success. Whether you prefer hearty oatmeal creations, protein-packed smoothie bowls, or egg-cellent breakfast ideas, there's a morning meal to suit every taste and dietary preference. So, rise and shine with these delicious and nutritious breakfast options, and get ready to tackle whatever the day throws your way with energy and vitality.

Simple and Delicious Breakfast Recipes

Starting your day with a nutritious breakfast is essential for maintaining optimal health, especially for individuals managing asthma. A wholesome breakfast not only provides the energy needed to kick start your day but also supports respiratory health, helping to alleviate asthma symptoms and promote better breathing. In this collection of simple and delicious breakfast recipes, we'll explore nourishing options that are both asthma-friendly and bursting with flavour, ensuring you start your day on the right note.

Berry Blast Smoothie Bowl:

Ingredients:

- 1 cup mixed berries (such as strawberries, blueberries, and raspberries)
- 1 ripe banana
- 1/2 cup Greek yogurt
- 1/4 cup almond milk
- Toppings: granola, sliced almonds, chia seeds, honey

Instructions:

- In a blender, combine the mixed berries, banana, Greek yogurt, and almond milk. Blend until smooth and creamy.
- Pour the smoothie into a bowl and top with granola, sliced almonds, chia seeds, and a drizzle of honey.
- Enjoy immediately with a spoon for a refreshing and nutritious breakfast that's rich in antioxidants and vitamins to support respiratory health.

Avocado and Egg Breakfast Bowl:

Ingredients:

- 1 ripe avocado
- 2 eggs
- Salt and pepper to taste
- 1 whole-grain English muffin (or bread of choice)

Instructions:

- Cut the avocado in half and remove the pit. Scoop out some of the flesh to create a well for the egg.
- Crack one egg into each avocado half.
- Season with salt and pepper.
- Place the avocado halves on a baking sheet and bake at 375°F (190°C) for 12-15 minutes, or until the eggs are set.
- Toast the English muffin or bread.
- Serve the baked avocado and eggs on top of the toasted English muffin or bread for a hearty and nutritious breakfast.

Apple Cinnamon Oatmeal:

- Ingredients:
- 1/2 cup rolled oats
- 1 cup water (or milk of choice)
- 1/2 apple, diced
- 1 tablespoon maple syrup (optional)
- 1/2 teaspoon cinnamon
- 1 tablespoon chopped nuts (almonds, walnuts, or pecans)

Instructions:

- In a saucepan, combine rolled oats and water (or milk) over medium heat.
- Stir in diced apple, maple syrup (if using), and cinnamon.
- Cook for 5-7 minutes, stirring occasionally, until the oats are tender and the mixture thickens.
- Remove from heat and transfer to a bowl.
- Sprinkle with chopped nuts for added crunch and protein.
- Enjoy this comforting and fibre-rich oatmeal to start your day on a wholesome note.

These simple and delicious breakfast recipes are not only satisfying and flavourful but also tailored to support asthma relief and overall well-being. By incorporating nutrient-rich ingredients like berries, avocado, eggs, and oats into your morning routine, you can fuel your body with the necessary nutrients to manage asthma symptoms and promote respiratory health. So, start your day right with these wholesome breakfast delights and enjoy the benefits of a nourishing meal for your body and mind.

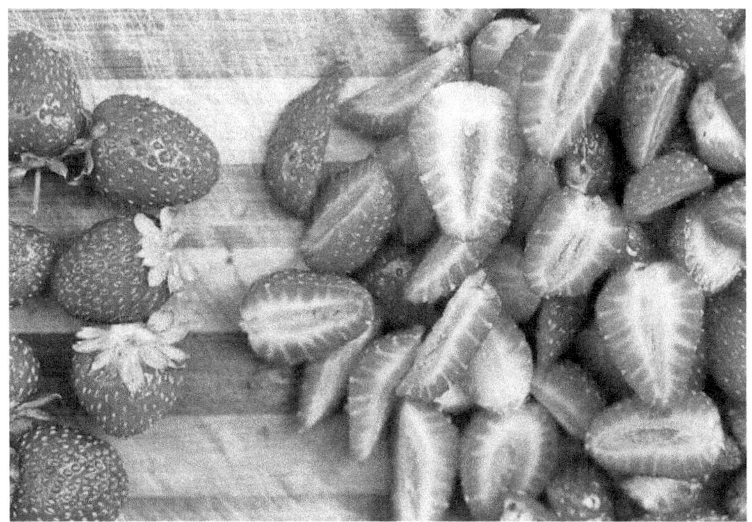

CHAPTER FIVE

Lung-Boosting Lunches

Lunchtime offers a golden opportunity to refuel your body with nutrients that support respiratory health and keep your energy levels high throughout the day. Incorporating lung-boosting ingredients into your midday meals can help optimize lung function and promote overall well-being.

Grilled Salmon Salad:

Grilled salmon is rich in omega-3 fatty acids, which have anti-inflammatory properties that support lung health. Pair it with a colorful salad made with leafy greens, tomatoes, cucumbers, and avocado for a nutrient-packed lunch that's as delicious as it is nutritious.

Quinoa and Vegetable Stir-Fry:

Quinoa is a complete protein and a good source of fiber, vitamins, and minerals, making it an excellent choice for a lung-boosting lunch. Stir-fry cooked quinoa with an assortment of colorful vegetables like bell peppers, broccoli, carrots, and snap peas in a flavorful sauce made with ginger, garlic, and soy sauce for a satisfying and nutritious meal.

Turkey and Avocado Wrap:

Turkey is a lean source of protein that provides essential nutrients like zinc and vitamin B6, which support immune function and respiratory health. Spread mashed avocado onto a whole-grain wrap, then layer on slices of roasted turkey breast, lettuce, tomato, and cucumber for a delicious and nutritious lunch option.

Vegetable and Lentil Soup:

Lentils are high in fiber and protein and are packed with nutrients like folate, iron, and magnesium, which support lung health. Combine cooked lentils with an assortment of vegetables like carrots, celery, onions, and spinach in a flavorful broth for a hearty and nourishing soup that's perfect for lunchtime.

Mediterranean Chickpea Salad:

Chickpeas are rich in fiber and protein and contain essential nutrients like folate and magnesium, which support lung function. Toss cooked chickpeas with diced tomatoes, cucumbers, red onions, Kalamata olives, and feta cheese in a lemon-herb vinaigrette for a refreshing and satisfying salad that's bursting with flavor and nutrition.

Spinach and Mushroom Quiche:

Spinach is rich in vitamins A and C, which have antioxidant properties that help protect lung cells from damage. Combine sautéed spinach and mushrooms with eggs, milk, and cheese in a whole-grain crust for a delicious and nutritious quiche that's perfect for lunch or dinner.

Incorporating lung-boosting ingredients into your midday meals is an effective way to support respiratory health and promote overall well-being. Whether you prefer grilled salmon salad, quinoa and vegetable stir-fry, turkey and avocado wrap, vegetable and lentil soup, Mediterranean chickpea salad, or spinach and mushroom quiche, there are plenty of delicious and nutritious lunch options to choose from. So, nourish your lungs with these nutrient-packed lunch ideas and enjoy the benefits of optimal respiratory health for years to come.

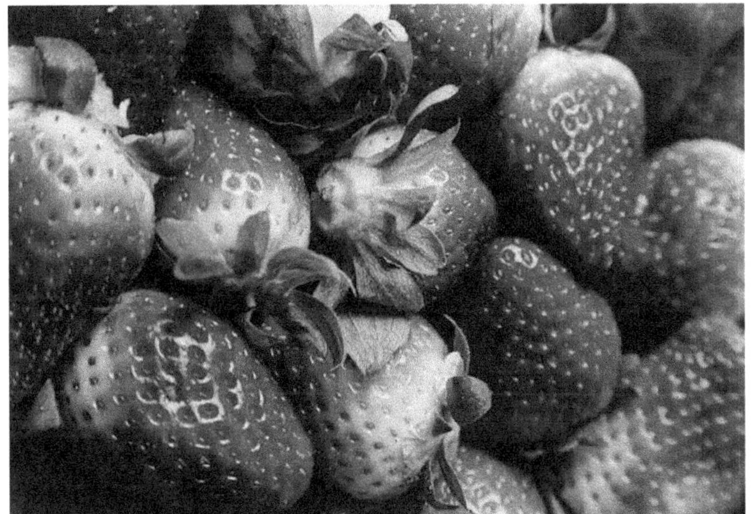

CHAPTER SIX

Breathing Easy Dinners

For individuals managing asthma, choosing the right foods for dinner and evening meals is crucial to support respiratory health and overall well-being. Dinner options that are rich in nutrients, low in potential triggers, and easy to digest can help asthma patients breathe easier and feel their best.

Grilled Salmon with Steamed Vegetables:

Grilled salmon is an excellent source of omega-3 fatty acids, which have anti-inflammatory properties that can help reduce airway inflammation in asthma patients. Serve grilled salmon with a side of steamed vegetables like broccoli, carrots, and zucchini for a nutritious and satisfying dinner that's easy on the lungs.

Quinoa and Black Bean Bowl:

Quinoa is a complete protein and a good source of fibre, vitamins, and minerals, making it an ideal choice for asthma patients. Combine cooked quinoa with black beans, diced tomatoes, avocado, and cilantro for a flavourful and filling dinner that's packed with nutrients and easy to digest.

Chicken and Vegetable Stir-Fry:

Lean protein sources like chicken breast are essential for muscle repair and respiratory health. Stir-fry sliced chicken breast with an assortment of colourful vegetables like bell peppers, snap peas, and mushrooms in a light sauce made with garlic, ginger, and low-sodium soy sauce. Serve over brown rice or cauliflower rice for a delicious and nutritious dinner option.

Vegetarian Lentil Soup:

Lentils are high in fibre and protein and contain essential nutrients like folate and magnesium, which support lung function. Combine cooked lentils with diced tomatoes, carrots, celery, onions, and spinach in a flavourful broth seasoned with cumin, coriander, and turmeric for a hearty and nourishing soup that's perfect for a comforting evening meal.

Baked Sweet Potato with Greek Yogurt and Broccoli:

Sweet potatoes are rich in beta-carotene and vitamin C, which have antioxidant properties that can help protect lung cells from damage. Bake sweet potatoes until tender, then top with a dollop of Greek yogurt and steamed broccoli for a simple yet satisfying dinner that's packed with nutrients and flavour.

Mushroom and Spinach Frittata:

Eggs are a nutrient-dense source of protein and essential vitamins and minerals, including vitamin D, which is important for respiratory health. Whip up a mushroom and spinach frittata by sautéing sliced mushrooms and spinach in a skillet, then pouring beaten eggs over the top and baking until set. Serve with a side salad for a nutritious and easy-to-make dinner option.

Choosing the right foods for dinner and evening meals is essential for asthma patients looking to optimize respiratory health and overall well-being.

By incorporating nutrient-rich ingredients like salmon, quinoa, chicken, lentils, sweet potatoes, and eggs into their meals, asthma patients can support lung function, reduce inflammation, and breathe easier. So, whip up one of these nutritious dinner ideas and enjoy the benefits of optimal respiratory health for years to come.

Family-Friendly Dinner Recipes

Baked Herb-Crusted Salmon with Roasted Vegetables:

Ingredients:

- 4 salmon fillets
- 2 tablespoons olive oil
- 1 tablespoon chopped fresh herbs (such as parsley, dill, or thyme)
- 1 teaspoon lemon zest
- Salt and pepper to taste
- Assorted vegetables (such as carrots, broccoli, and bell peppers), chopped

Instructions:

1. Preheat the oven to 400°F (200°C).
2. Place the salmon fillets on a baking sheet lined with parchment paper.

3. In a small bowl, mix together olive oil, chopped herbs, lemon zest, salt, and pepper.

4. Brush the herb mixture over the salmon fillets.

5. Arrange the chopped vegetables around the salmon on the baking sheet.

6. Bake for 15-20 minutes, or until the salmon is cooked through and the vegetables are tender.

7. Serve the herb-crusted salmon with roasted vegetables for a flavorful and nutritious dinner that's rich in omega-3 fatty acids and antioxidants.

Turkey and Vegetable Quinoa Skillet:

Ingredients:

- 1 tablespoon olive oil
- 1 pound ground turkey
- 1 onion, diced
- 2 cloves garlic, minced
- 1 bell pepper, diced
- 1 zucchini, diced
- 1 cup quinoa, rinsed
- 2 cups low-sodium chicken broth

- 1 teaspoon smoked paprika
- Salt and pepper to taste
- Chopped fresh parsley for garnish

Instructions:

1. Heat olive oil in a large skillet over medium heat.
2. Add ground turkey to the skillet and cook until browned, breaking it up with a spoon as it cooks.
3. Add diced onion, minced garlic, bell pepper, and zucchini to the skillet. Cook until vegetables are tender, about 5-7 minutes.
4. Stir in quinoa, chicken broth, smoked paprika, salt, and pepper. Bring to a boil.
5. Reduce heat to low, cover, and simmer for 15-20 minutes, or until quinoa is cooked and liquid is absorbed.
6. Fluff quinoa with a fork and garnish with chopped fresh parsley before serving.
7. Enjoy this protein-packed and fiber-rich turkey and vegetable quinoa skillet for a satisfying family dinner that's both nutritious and delicious.

Vegetable and Lentil Soup:

Ingredients:

- 1 tablespoon olive oil
- 1 onion, diced
- 2 carrots, diced
- 2 celery stalks, diced
- 2 cloves garlic, minced
- 1 cup dried green lentils, rinsed
- 6 cups low-sodium vegetable broth
- 1 bay leaf
- 1 teaspoon dried thyme
- Salt and pepper to taste
- Chopped fresh parsley for garnish

Instructions:

1. Heat olive oil in a large pot over medium heat.
2. Add diced onion, carrots, celery, and minced garlic to the pot. Cook until vegetables are softened, about 5-7 minutes.
3. Stir in dried green lentils, vegetable broth, bay leaf, dried thyme, salt, and pepper. Bring to a boil.

4. Reduce heat to low, cover, and simmer for 30-40 minutes, or until lentils are tender.

5. Remove bay leaf from the soup and discard.

6. Ladle soup into bowls and garnish with chopped fresh parsley before serving.

7. Serve this hearty and nutritious vegetable and lentil soup with crusty bread for a comforting family dinner that's perfect for chilly evenings.

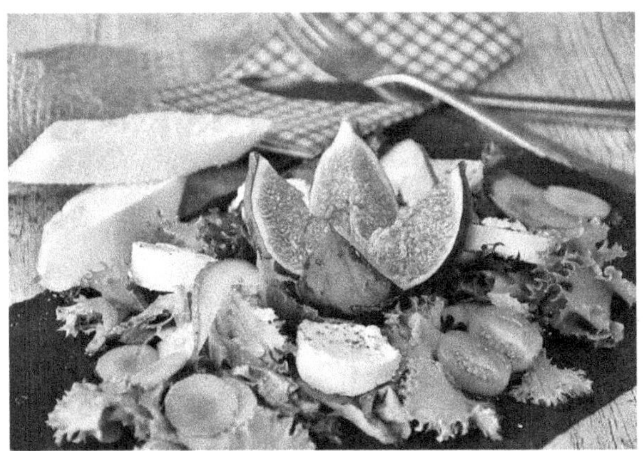

CHAPTER SEVEN

Smart Snacks and Smoothies For Asthma Relief

Snacks

Snacking plays a significant role in maintaining energy levels and supporting overall well-being, especially for individuals managing asthma. Smart snacks for asthma relief prioritize nutrient-dense ingredients that can help reduce inflammation, support lung function, and provide sustained energy throughout the day.

Apple Slices with Almond Butter:

Apples are rich in antioxidants and vitamin C, which can help reduce inflammation in the airways. Pairing apple slices with almond butter adds healthy fats and protein, providing a satisfying and nutritious snack that can help stabilize blood sugar levels and keep energy levels steady.

Greek Yogurt with Berries and Honey:

Greek yogurt is an excellent source of protein and pro-biotics, which support immune function and gut health. Top Greek yogurt with fresh berries like blueberries, strawberries, or raspberries, and drizzle with a touch of honey for a sweet and creamy snack that's rich in antioxidants and vitamins.

Mixed Nuts and Dried Fruit:

A mix of nuts and dried fruit provides a balanced combination of protein, healthy fats, and fiber, making it an ideal snack for asthma relief. Choose unsalted nuts like almonds, walnuts, or pistachios, and pair them with dried fruit like apricots, raisins, or cranberries for a satisfying and nutritious snack that can help keep hunger at bay.

Carrot Sticks with Hummus:

Carrots are rich in beta-carotene and vitamin A, which have antioxidant properties that can help protect lung cells from damage. Pair carrot sticks with hummus for a crunchy and satisfying snack that's packed with vitamins, minerals, and fiber, supporting respiratory health and overall well-being.

Avocado Toast with Whole-Grain Bread:

Avocado is rich in healthy fats and fiber, which can help reduce inflammation and support lung function. Spread mashed avocado onto whole-grain toast for a delicious and nutritious snack that's rich in vitamins, minerals, and antioxidants, providing sustained energy and promoting respiratory health.

Edamame Beans:

Edamame beans are a good source of plant-based protein and fiber, making them an excellent snack option for individuals with asthma. Enjoy edamame beans on their own or sprinkle them with a touch of sea salt and black pepper for a savory and satisfying snack that's rich in nutrients and supports respiratory health.

Refreshing Smoothie Recipes

Green Goddess Smoothie:

Ingredients:

- 1 cup spinach
- 1/2 cup kale
- 1/2 cucumber, peeled
- 1/2 green apple, cored
- 1/2 banana
- 1 tablespoon chia seeds
- 1 cup coconut water

Instructions:

1.	Add all ingredients to a blender and blend until smooth.
2.	Pour into a glass and enjoy this refreshing green smoothie packed with vitamins, minerals, and antioxidants to support respiratory health.

Berry Blast Smoothie:

Ingredients:

- 1/2 cup mixed berries (strawberries, blueberries, raspberries)
- 1/2 banana
- 1/2 cup Greek yogurt
- 1 tablespoon honey
- 1/2 cup almond milk

Instructions:

1.   Combine all ingredients in a blender and blend until smooth.

2.   Pour into a glass and enjoy this antioxidant-rich smoothie that's perfect for asthma relief and overall well-being.

Tropical Turmeric Smoothie:

Ingredients:

- 1/2 cup pineapple chunks
- 1/2 banana
- 1/2 teaspoon turmeric
- 1/2 teaspoon ginger
- 1 tablespoon honey
- 1/2 cup coconut water

Instructions:

1.   Place all ingredients in a blender and blend until smooth.
2.   Pour into a glass and savor this tropical smoothie with anti-inflammatory properties to support respiratory health.

CHAPTER EIGHT

Herbal Helpers and Natural Remedies

Asthma is a chronic respiratory condition characterized by airway inflammation, broncho constriction, and increased mucus production. Managing asthma typically involves prescribed medications, but many individuals seek complementary and alternative therapies to support their respiratory health. It is crucial to consult with a healthcare professional before integrating these remedies into your routine, particularly if you have a chronic condition like asthma.

Beneficial Herbs for Asthma

Ginger (Zingiber officinale)

- Benefits: Anti-inflammatory properties help relax the airways.
- How to Use: Ginger tea, fresh ginger in food, or ginger supplements.

Turmeric (Curcuma longa)

- Benefits: Contains curcumin, which has anti-inflammatory and antioxidant properties.
- How to Use: Turmeric tea, golden milk, or turmeric supplements.

Licorice Root (Glycyrrhiza glabra)

- Benefits: Acts as an expectorant and has anti-inflammatory properties.
- How to Use: Licorice tea or licorice root supplements. Note: Not recommended for prolonged use or for people with high blood pressure.

Thyme (Thymus vulgaris)

- Benefits: Acts as a natural expectorant, helps in mucus clearance.
- How to Use: Thyme tea, adding thyme to food, or thyme oil inhalation.

Mullein (Verbascum thapsus)

- Benefits: Soothes the respiratory tract and reduces inflammation.
- How to Use: Mullein tea or mullein leaf tincture.

Peppermint (Mentha piperita)

- Benefits: Contains menthol which helps in opening up airways.
- How to Use: Peppermint tea or inhaling peppermint essential oil (diluted).

Safe and Effective Natural Remedies

Steam Inhalation

- Benefits: Helps in loosening mucus and opening airways.
- How to Use: Boil water, pour it into a bowl, lean over it with a towel over your head, and inhale the steam. Adding a few drops of eucalyptus or peppermint oil can enhance effectiveness.

Honey

- Benefits: Soothes the throat and can act as a natural cough suppressant.
- How to Use: Mix honey in warm water or herbal tea and drink it.

Omega-3 Fatty Acids

- Benefits: Reduces inflammation and may improve lung function.
- How to Use: Include sources like flaxseeds, chia seeds, walnuts, and fatty fish in your diet or take omega-3 supplements.

Breathing Exercises

- Benefits: Helps in strengthening respiratory muscles and improving lung function.
- How to Use: Practice techniques such as diaphragmatic breathing, pursed-lip breathing, or the Buteyko method.

Acupuncture

- Benefits: May help in reducing asthma symptoms and improving lung function.
- How to Use: Seek treatment from a licensed acupuncturist.

Dietary Changes

- Benefits: Reduces inflammation and prevents asthma triggers.
- How to Use: Incorporate anti-inflammatory foods such as leafy greens, berries, nuts, and seeds. Avoid potential triggers like dairy, processed foods, and allergens.

Important Notes

Consistency: Regular use of these remedies can help manage symptoms, but they are not substitutes for prescribed asthma medications.

Allergies: Be aware of any potential allergies to herbs or natural substances.

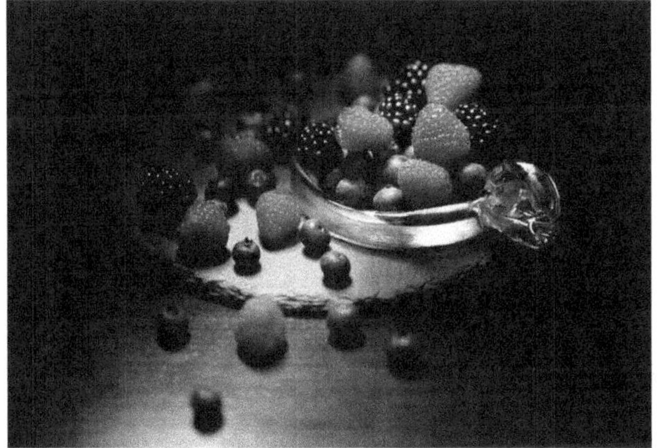

CHAPTER NINE

Meal Planning for Better Breathing

Asthma, a chronic respiratory condition characterized by inflammation and narrowing of the airways, affects millions of people worldwide. While medications and medical treatments are essential for managing asthma, dietary choices can also play a significant role in alleviating symptoms and improving overall lung function. This chapter explores the principles of meal planning for better breathing, provides weekly meal plans designed to support asthma relief, and offers tips for efficient meal prep.

Research suggests that certain foods and nutrients can influence inflammation and lung function, making diet an important factor in managing asthma. An anti-inflammatory diet, rich in fruits, vegetables, whole grains, and healthy fats, can help reduce airway inflammation and improve respiratory health. Conversely, processed foods, high-sugar snacks, and food allergens can exacerbate asthma symptoms.

Weekly Meal Plans for Asthma Relief

To support respiratory health, the following meal plans focus on nutrient-dense foods known for their anti-inflammatory properties and ability to support lung function.

Week 1

Monday:

- Breakfast: Oatmeal topped with fresh berries, flaxseeds, and a drizzle of honey.
- Lunch: Quinoa salad with chickpeas, cherry tomatoes, cucumbers, and a lemon-tahini dressing.
- Dinner: Grilled salmon with steamed broccoli and sweet potato.

Tuesday:

- Breakfast: Smoothie with spinach, banana, almond milk, and chia seeds.
- Lunch: Lentil soup with mixed greens and a whole grain roll.
- Dinner: Stir-fried tofu with mixed vegetables (bell peppers, carrots, snap peas) over brown rice.

Wednesday:

- Breakfast: Greek yogurt with walnuts, honey, and sliced strawberries.
- Lunch: Turkey and avocado wrap with a side of mixed greens.
- Dinner: Baked chicken breast with quinoa and roasted Brussels sprouts.

Thursday:

- Breakfast: Whole grain toast with mashed avocado and a poached egg.
- Lunch: Spinach and kale salad with grilled chicken, apple slices, walnuts, and a balsamic vinaigrette.

- Dinner: Vegetable curry with chickpeas, served over basmati rice.

Friday:

- Breakfast: Smoothie bowl with blended acai, topped with granola, coconut flakes, and blueberries.
- Lunch: Mediterranean bowl with falafel, hummus, tabbouleh, and mixed greens.
- Dinner: Grilled shrimp with zucchini noodles and cherry tomato salad.

Saturday:

- Breakfast: Chia seed pudding with almond milk, topped with mango and pistachios.
- Lunch: Brown rice and black bean burrito bowl with salsa, guacamole, and mixed greens.
- Dinner: Baked cod with quinoa, roasted carrots, and a side of steamed spinach.

Sunday:

- Breakfast: Scrambled eggs with spinach, tomatoes, and feta cheese.
- Lunch: Butternut squash soup with a side of arugula salad.
- Dinner: Turkey meatballs with whole grain pasta and marinara sauce.

Week 2

Monday:

- Breakfast: Overnight oats with almond milk, chia seeds, and fresh raspberries.
- Lunch: Chicken and vegetable stir-fry with quinoa.
- Dinner: Baked trout with roasted sweet potatoes and green beans.

Tuesday:

- Breakfast: Smoothie with kale, pineapple, coconut water, and flaxseed.
- Lunch: Mixed bean salad with avocado, cherry tomatoes, and lime dressing.
- Dinner: Turkey chili with a side of cornbread.

Wednesday:

- Breakfast: Cottage cheese with sliced peaches and sunflower seeds.
- Lunch: Whole grain pita with hummus, grilled vegetables, and a side of mixed greens.
- Dinner: Lentil and vegetable stew with a side of brown rice.

Thursday:

- Breakfast: Whole grain waffles topped with Greek yogurt and blueberries.
- Lunch: Quinoa and kale salad with pomegranate seeds, walnuts, and a citrus vinaigrette.

- Dinner: Baked chicken thighs with roasted parsnips and a side of sauted spinach.

Friday:

- Breakfast: Smoothie bowl with blended spinach, kiwi, and banana, topped with granola.
- Lunch: Grilled salmon salad with mixed greens, cherry tomatoes, cucumber, and olive oil dressing.
- Dinner: Vegetable lasagna with whole grain noodles and a side of steamed broccoli.

Saturday:

- Breakfast: Chia seed pudding with coconut milk, topped with fresh berries and almonds.
- Lunch: Black bean and sweet potato tacos with avocado and cilantro.
- Dinner: Baked cod with a quinoa and black bean salad.

Sunday:

- Breakfast: Scrambled tofu with mushrooms, spinach, and bell peppers.
- Lunch: Tomato and basil soup with a side of whole grain bread.
- Dinner: Stuffed bell peppers with ground turkey, quinoa, and mixed vegetables.

Tips for Efficient Meal Prep

Efficient meal prep can save time and ensure that you have healthy meals ready to support your asthma management. Here are some tips to make meal prep more effective:

- Create a weekly meal plan and shopping list. This reduces last-minute grocery trips and helps you stick to a healthy eating routine.
- Cook large batches of grains (quinoa, brown rice) and proteins (chicken, tofu) at the beginning of the week. Portion them into individual servings for quick meals.

- Wash, chop, and store vegetables in airtight containers in the refrigerator. This makes it easy to assemble salads, stir-fries, and snacks.

- Prepare and freeze meals like soups, stews, and casseroles. These can be reheated quickly for a nutritious meal when time is limited.

- Prepare healthy snacks in advance, such as sliced fruits, nuts, and yogurt. This ensures you have asthma-friendly options available between meals.

- Use glass containers for meal storage to keep food fresh and reduce exposure to plastic chemicals that can be harmful to health.

- Rotate different recipes and ingredients to ensure you get a wide range of nutrients and avoid meal fatigue.

- Prepare infused water with fruits and herbs to encourage hydration, which is crucial for respiratory health.

Meal planning for better breathing involves incorporating anti-inflammatory foods and avoiding potential asthma triggers. By following the weekly meal plans provided and implementing efficient meal prep strategies, individuals with asthma can support their respiratory health and improve their overall well-being. Remember to consult with a healthcare professional or a nutritionist to tailor dietary choices to your specific needs and ensure they complement your medical treatment for asthma.

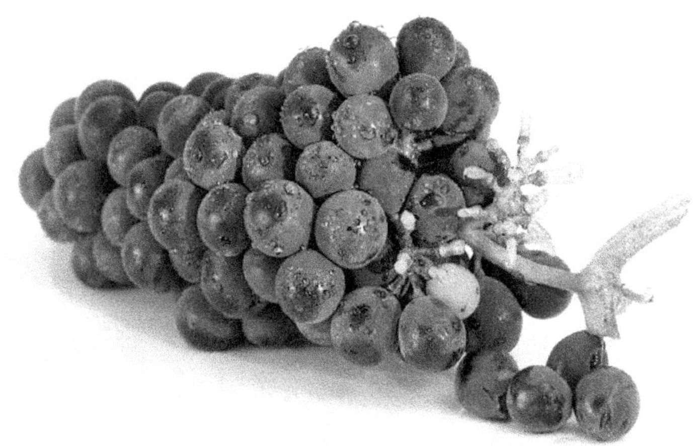

CHAPTER TEN

Real-Life Success Stories

Asthma is a chronic condition that can significantly impact daily life, but many individuals have found ways to manage their symptoms effectively and lead fulfilling lives. Real-life success stories offer hope and practical advice to others facing similar challenges.

Inspiring Stories of Asthma Management

1. Emily's Journey to Breathable Freedom

Emily, a 35-year-old teacher from New York, was diagnosed with asthma at the age of 10. Her asthma was triggered by allergens and cold weather, making it difficult for her to participate in outdoor activities. For years, Emily relied heavily on inhalers and avoided strenuous activities. However, a turning point came when she decided to take control of her health through lifestyle changes.

Emily began practicing yoga and meditation to manage stress, which she noticed significantly reduced her asthma flare-ups. She also revamped her diet, incorporating more anti-inflammatory foods like leafy greens, berries, and omega-3 rich fish. Additionally, she started using a humidifier during the winter months to keep the air in her home moist, reducing the frequency of her attacks.

Today, Emily enjoys hiking and even completed a 5K race. She continues to practice yoga and maintains a healthy diet, attributing these changes to her improved asthma management.

2. Jake's Athletic Triumph

Jake, a 22-year-old college student and avid soccer player from California, faced severe asthma that often interrupted his athletic pursuits. Determined not to let asthma define him, Jake worked closely with his pulmonologist and a sports trainer to develop a personalized asthma action plan.

This plan included a warm-up routine designed to prepare his lungs for physical activity, using a pre-exercise inhaler, and recognizing early signs of an asthma attack. Jake also paid attention to environmental triggers, avoiding outdoor practice during high pollen days or extreme temperatures.

With these strategies, Jake managed to keep his asthma under control and eventually became the captain of his college soccer team. He now inspires his teammates and others with asthma to pursue their passions with determination and proper management.

3. Lisa's Path to Natural Remedies

Lisa, a 40-year-old mother from Texas, struggled with asthma symptoms that often interfered with her busy life. Frustrated with frequent medication adjustments, Lisa turned to natural remedies and holistic approaches to supplement her asthma management.

She explored various herbs known for their respiratory benefits, such as ginger, turmeric, and licorice root. Incorporating these into her daily routine, along with essential oils like eucalyptus for steam inhalation, Lisa experienced a noticeable improvement in her symptoms.

Lisa also prioritized a clean home environment, reducing dust and mold through regular cleaning and using air purifiers. These changes, combined with her prescribed medication, helped Lisa achieve a better quality of life and manage her asthma more effectively.

Practical Tips from Asthma Warriors

The following practical tips from asthma warriors like Emily, Jake, and Lisa can help others manage their asthma more effectively:

1. Develop a Personalized Asthma Action Plan

Work with your healthcare provider to create a detailed asthma action plan tailored to your specific triggers and symptoms.

Include instructions for daily management, medication use, and steps to take during an asthma attack.

2. Identify and Avoid Triggers

Keep a diary to track asthma symptoms and identify potential triggers such as allergens, weather changes, and stress.

Minimize exposure to known triggers by making environmental modifications, such as using air purifiers, avoiding smoking areas, and keeping windows closed during high pollen seasons.

3. Incorporate Regular Exercise

Engage in regular physical activity to strengthen respiratory muscles and improve lung function. Choose asthma-friendly exercises like swimming, walking, or yoga.

Always warm up before exercising and use a pre-exercise inhaler if prescribed by your doctor.

4. Practice Breathing Techniques

Learn and practice breathing techniques such as diaphragmatic breathing and pursed-lip breathing to improve lung capacity and reduce asthma symptoms.

Consider joining a pulmonary rehabilitation program to receive professional guidance on effective breathing exercises.

5. Maintain a Healthy Diet

Adopt an anti-inflammatory diet rich in fruits, vegetables, whole grains, and healthy fats to support overall respiratory health.

Avoid processed foods, high-sugar snacks, and known food allergens that can exacerbate asthma symptoms.

6. Manage Stress and Mental Health

Practice stress-reduction techniques such as yoga, meditation, or mindfulness to lower the risk of stress-induced asthma attacks.

Seek support from friends, family, or a therapist to manage anxiety and depression related to asthma.

7. Stay Informed and Connected

Educate yourself about asthma through reliable sources and stay updated on new treatments and management strategies.

Join asthma support groups or online communities to connect with others who understand your challenges and can offer advice and encouragement.

Real-life success stories of asthma management showcase the resilience and determination of individuals who have found effective ways to live well with their condition. By sharing their journeys and practical tips, these asthma warriors provide valuable insights and inspiration to others facing similar challenges.

Remember, asthma management is a continuous process, and with the right strategies and support, it is possible to lead a healthy and active life. Always consult with healthcare professionals to tailor these tips to your specific needs and ensure they complement your prescribed treatment plan.

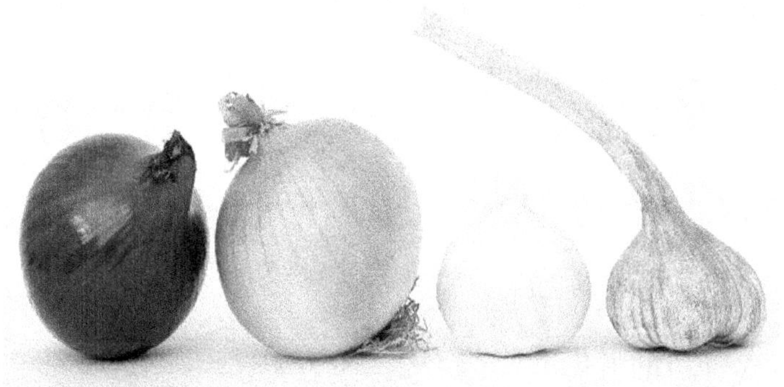

CHAPTER ELEVEN

Sustainable Eating for Long-Term Relief

Managing chronic conditions such as asthma through diet requires a sustainable approach that not only provides relief from symptoms but also promotes overall health and well-being. Sustainable eating involves making consistent, healthful food choices that can be maintained over the long term.

Maintaining a Balanced Diet

A balanced diet is foundational to sustainable eating and can significantly impact asthma management. It involves consuming a variety of foods that provide essential nutrients needed for optimal health and reduced inflammation. Here are key components to consider:

1. Incorporate Anti-Inflammatory Foods

Chronic inflammation is a hallmark of asthma, and certain foods can help reduce this inflammation:

Fruits and Vegetables: Rich in antioxidants and vitamins, fruits and vegetables help combat inflammation. Aim to include a variety of colors to ensure a broad spectrum of nutrients. Berries, leafy greens, bell peppers, and citrus fruits are particularly beneficial.

Healthy Fats: Omega-3 fatty acids, found in fatty fish (such as salmon and mackerel), flaxseeds, chia seeds, and walnuts, have strong anti-inflammatory properties.

Whole Grains: Whole grains like brown rice, quinoa, and oats provide fiber and essential nutrients that support overall health.

Herbs and Spices: Turmeric, ginger, garlic, and cinnamon have anti-inflammatory and antioxidant properties. Incorporating these into your meals can add flavor and health benefits.

2. Avoid Potential Triggers

Certain foods can exacerbate asthma symptoms in some individuals. Identifying and avoiding these triggers can help manage asthma more effectively:

Processed Foods: High in preservatives, artificial additives, and unhealthy fats, processed foods can increase inflammation and should be minimized.

Dairy Products: For some people, dairy can trigger asthma symptoms. If you suspect dairy may be a trigger, consider alternatives like almond, soy, or oat milk.

Sulfites: Commonly found in dried fruits, wine, and processed foods, sulfites can trigger asthma attacks in sensitive individuals.

Food Allergens: Common allergens like nuts, shellfish, and gluten can exacerbate asthma symptoms. Be mindful of any personal food sensitivities or allergies.

3. Stay Hydrated

Proper hydration is crucial for maintaining mucus consistency in the airways and supporting overall lung function. Aim to drink at least 8 glasses of water per day, and consider herbal teas and water-rich fruits and vegetables (like cucumbers and melons) as additional sources of hydration.

4. Balance Macronutrients

Ensure your diet includes a balance of carbohydrates, proteins, and fats to provide sustained energy and support bodily functions:

Carbohydrates: Focus on complex carbohydrates such as whole grains, legumes, and vegetables, which provide long-lasting energy and fiber.

Proteins: Incorporate lean protein sources such as poultry, fish, beans, and legumes to support muscle maintenance and repair.

Fats: Include healthy fats from sources like avocados, nuts, seeds, and olive oil, which are essential for hormone production and nutrient absorption.

Adapting Your Diet Over Time

Sustainable eating is not a static process but one that evolves with your changing needs, preferences, and health status. Here are strategies to adapt your diet over time:

1. Monitor and Adjust

Regularly track your diet and asthma symptoms to identify patterns and make necessary adjustments. A food diary can help you pinpoint which foods may be triggering symptoms and which provide relief.

Elimination Diet: If you suspect certain foods are worsening your asthma, try an elimination diet to systematically identify and remove potential triggers. Reintroduce foods one at a time to observe any reactions.

Seasonal Adjustments: Adjust your diet according to seasonal changes. For example, in winter, you might increase your intake of vitamin D-rich foods like fatty fish and fortified cereals to compensate for reduced sunlight exposure.

2. Incorporate New Foods Gradually

Introduce new, healthy foods gradually to ensure they suit your preferences and digestive system. This approach helps maintain variety in your diet without causing abrupt changes that might lead to nutritional imbalances.

3. Stay Informed

Keep up-to-date with the latest research on nutrition and asthma management. Dietary recommendations can evolve based on new scientific findings, so staying informed helps you make evidence-based choices.

4. Seek Professional Guidance

Consult with healthcare professionals such as a registered dietitian or nutritionist to tailor your diet to your specific needs. They can provide personalized advice and help you navigate dietary changes effectively.

5. Balance Convenience with Health

Life can be busy, and convenience is key to maintaining a sustainable diet. Plan and prepare meals in advance to ensure you have healthy options available even during hectic times. Utilize tools like meal prepping, batch cooking, and freezing healthy meals.

Practical Tips for Sustainable Eating

Here are some additional practical tips to help you maintain a sustainable, balanced diet:

Cook at Home: Home-cooked meals give you control over ingredients and cooking methods, helping you avoid hidden allergens and unhealthy additives.

Experiment with Recipes: Keep your meals interesting by trying new recipes and cooking techniques. This can prevent dietary fatigue and ensure you enjoy your food.

Grow Your Own: If possible, grow your own herbs, vegetables, or fruits. This can be a rewarding way to ensure fresh, organic produce is readily available.

Educate Yourself: Learn about nutrition labels and how to read them effectively. Understanding what goes into your food helps you make healthier choices.

Mindful Eating: Practice mindful eating by paying attention to your hunger and fullness cues, savoring your food, and avoiding distractions while eating. This can improve digestion and satisfaction with your meals.

Sustainable eating for long-term relief involves maintaining a balanced diet rich in anti-inflammatory foods, avoiding potential triggers, and making adaptive changes over time. By incorporating these principles into your daily routine, you can manage asthma symptoms more effectively and promote overall health and well-being. Remember, a sustainable diet is not about perfection but about making consistent, healthful choices that support your long-term health goals. Always consult with healthcare professionals to tailor your diet to your specific needs and ensure it complements your overall asthma management plan.

CONCLUSION

As we reach the conclusion of "ASTHMA-WHOLESOME EATS: Nourishing Recipes for Lasting Relief," it's clear that the journey to easier breathing is a blend of informed choices, consistent effort, and a commitment to your well-being. This book has provided you with a variety of delicious, asthma-friendly recipes and practical dietary advice designed to support your respiratory health and enhance your overall quality of life.

By embracing the principles of sustainable eating and incorporating nutrient-dense, anti-inflammatory foods into your daily routine, you have taken significant steps toward managing your asthma more effectively. The recipes and tips shared in these pages are not just about temporary relief but about fostering lasting, positive changes that will benefit you for years to come.

Your journey to easier breathing is a continuous one, marked by ongoing learning and adaptation. Keep exploring new foods, experimenting with recipes, and refining your diet to suit your evolving needs. Remember, each small, mindful choice you make contributes to a healthier, more vibrant you.

We hope this book has inspired you and provided the tools you need to take control of your asthma through nourishing, wholesome eating. Here's to a future of flavourful meals, better breathing, and a life filled with vitality and joy.

Thank you for allowing us to be part of your journey. May your path to wellness be as fulfilling and rewarding as the meals you've prepared and enjoyed.

As you close this book, know that your journey to easier breathing and better health is just beginning. Continue to explore, learn, and thrive. Here's to your health, happiness, and the delicious journey ahead!